TACTICAL FITNESS

MANIFESTO

BY

Derek Zahler

TABLE OF CONTENTS

Introduction

Welcome to the Tactical Fitness Manifesto. These pages contain my methodology on physical training for athletes and professionals in the tactical fitness industry. The book is directed to strength & conditioning professionals, athletes, fitness retailers, tactical unit administrators and even the uninitiated - but curious - casual reader. Please keep an open mind and a motivated perspective.

While many elite fitness and nutrition experts have contributed to my experience and understanding of the field, this handbook represents my own unique perspective. I will defend, promote and explain my thoughts anecdotally. In the end, my goal is to enable others to build and develop their own methodologies using mine as a foundation. I want to initiate the kind of discussion that will create a productive and integrative landscape for athletes and coaches alike.

Tactical operators belong to a special group of athletes with unique needs tied to a variety of issues. It is irresponsible to treat the tactical athlete as a monolithic subset of traditional athletics.

What qualifies me to write this handbook? Quite simply, I care.

Beyond that, here is some background on my own experiences. In early 2002, I was looking forward to graduating from the University of California, Berkeley. As a member of both the boxing and football programs, I felt I had a good understanding of the role strength & conditioning programs play in athletic performance. Yes, I enjoyed competing in front of thousands of excited fans; however, I most appreciated the emotional toughness and mental focus that was sharpened through hours in the weight room.

The 9/11 attacks had occurred earlier in my senior year. I know I do not need to rehash the events of that day for anyone reading this, but it is probably worthwhile to mention that my increased feelings of patriotism and desire to participate in the U.S. response was overwhelming — but not necessarily shared by my classmates and professors.

Shortly after graduating in the spring of 2002, I took my able body, enlisted in the U.S. Army and started on the path to becoming a Special Forces operator. After 16 months of training, I was assigned to the 1st Special Forces Group in Okinawa, Japan (1-1 SFG) and served as the intelligence sergeant (MOS 18F) on an Operational Detachment Alpha (ODA), combat-dive team.

Through the years on ODA, I was given a variety of opportunities to test and sharpen the physical, mental and emotional skills I had acquired during my athletics career. And back then, I definitely had a bit of an ego about my physical abilities. After all, I had been a Division I athlete, right?

These days I look back at my training with the eyes of experience. The Combat Diver Qualification Course (CDQC) and Ranger School, were some of the most challenging physical tests I had ever been put through. Demanding more than physical readiness, these courses would test my mental and emotional character. Special Forces soldiers are more than physically fit animals; they are the manifestation of mental and emotional determination. Mind over matter, friend. If you don't mind, it don't matter.

I liked that idea, and I knew that

difficult things did not accomplish themselves. So, in 2009, I separated from active military duty and joined the civilian workforce. My plan was to leverage what I knew best — physical conditioning — into a successful career. I investigated and studied existing material and programs on physical fitness. I quickly learned that the training I had undergone in the Army — even in Special Forces — was not so special. High volume, high intensity, and low rest intervals encompass the entire military training philosophy for physical fitness.

At the time of this printing:
- There is only one Army Physical Fitness Test (APFT).
- There are over 250 Military Occupational Specialties (MOS).
- There are over 500,000 active Army soldiers.

Of course certain aspects of training

are uniform and so in certain ways, this makes sense. Components such as mental discipline, uniform metrics and emotional conditioning should be consistent for all soldiers so it is appropriate that the Army methodology would be universal in those areas. However, this mindset does not take into consideration the variety of body types, athletic backgrounds and operational demands that deserve special attention when physical conditioning is prescribed and executed.

I became determined to create better strength & conditioning programs for military personnel, with particular consideration for my former teammates who were still serving.

I began listening and thinking.

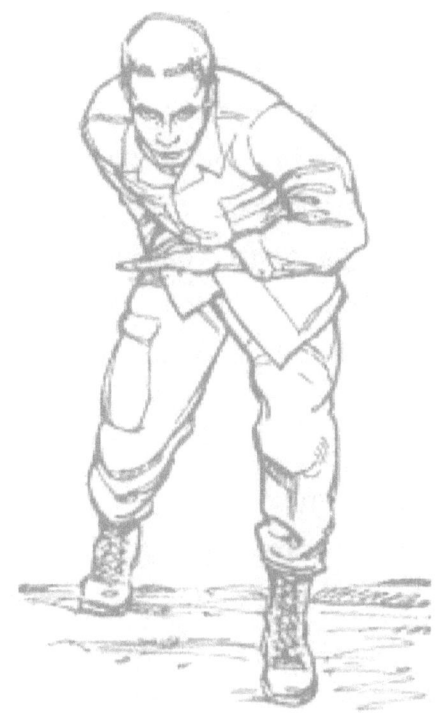

Section 1 – The Tactical Athlete

I define Tactical Athletes as: *People who use their bodies in a professional capacity to protect and/or secure themselves or others.*

The cornerstone of any strength & conditioning program should be to first analyze the individual athlete in order to construct the most appropriate program for that person. Unfortunately, the idea of specificity within programs has been lost in the current fitness climate.

The need for specificity is discussed in the publications of prominent educators and personalities; and yes, they appear sincere. However, most educators and celebrity-type personalities in the industry are extremely quick to completely omit the step of defining the athlete precisely, and instead, focus on highlighting unique modalities, introducing niche or boutique communities, emphasizing focused research, promoting special competitions and endorsing new - and generally expensive - equipment.

The goal of this manual is not to deconstruct or minimize the importance of modalities, nutritional programming or equipment selection. The goal here is to highlight the primary and most important facet of a good fitness program — attention to the individual athlete.

This is a publication on Tactical Fitness. Therefore, the athlete referred to in these pages is the "tactical athlete" (TA).

The common definition of the word "tactical" is: relating to, or constituting actions carefully planned to gain a specific operational outcome.

To begin, the TA will be defined anecdotally through professions. The core tactical professions are:

- Military
- Law Enforcement
- First Responder (including firefighters and paramedics)

These core groups encompasses key demographics or sub-groups that include, but are not limited to:

- Military veterans and recruits;
- Retired law enforcement officers and first responders; and,
- Medically disabled operators in any of the above fields.

Analyzing these professions provides a better understanding of the large mission scope of the tactical athlete. Moreover, it is easy to see how each of the fundamental groups may be broken into smaller ones. For example, it is possible to divide the military soldier group into combat and support operations, then military branches, and then operational specialties (e.g. direct action, recognizance and surveillance, etc.).

Once it is acknowledged that it is inappropriate to over-simplify classification of the tactical athlete into broad groups — such as all military personnel or all law enforcement officers -- we begin to understand the deficiencies in the programming and protocols that many educators currently promote. For example, it should not be assumed that all military personnel benefit from a protocol that promotes high volume anaerobic conditioning and power development.

A military sniper requires a very efficient cardiovascular system reliant on slower metabolic rates and greater aerobic capacity in order to perform longer, sustained missions in austere environments.

The implementation of Speed, Agility and Quickness (SAQ) protocol must also be carefully weighed. It is true that most tactical athletes possess a significant need for the development of dynamic movement in space. A degree of quickness and agility are paramount to accomplishing a variety of movements. However, it is very easy to fail the tactical athlete by focusing too much upon SAQ.

Most strength & conditioning professionals know that balance (joint stabilization) and core strength provide the foundation for any functionally fit athlete. And, muscular imbalances, synergistic dominance and postural deficiencies must be addressed in order for functional fitness to be achieved.

It is also well known that continued attention to core strength greatly supports and improves all movement and general wellness in athletes.

So, why do so many coaches and trainers skip the foundation of strength training and jump right into the power developments cycle?

Why waste so much time developing a type of fitness that is rarely used and ignore the facets of fitness that will keep an athlete functional?

It seems like a good idea to back up and ask: "Why do most strength & conditioning professionals prioritize power and strength development over stability and functional movement?" The answer is simple — Ego runs the industry.

It is boring and un-sexy to train on capacity and stability. Strength & conditioning professionals feel pressure to create niche markets in the industry by introducing "new" and fashionable concepts that produce athletes achieving remarkable numbers — and little else. These professionals are not focusing on the best interests of their athletes; they are working to achieve personal recognition in the field by attempting to differentiate themselves from everyone else out there.

This is a marketing game where these trainers are too absorbed in the idea of becoming the "winner" of the largest market share instead of providing the best possible services and programming to their athletes.

Those playing this game need to get out of the field as they are undermining the industry as a whole and failing athletes.

Most fitness educators include capacity development, strength promotion and power creation in their basic curriculum.

Elements of technique refinement and corrective exercise also accompany most entry-level programs. This leads to the question: Where is the disconnect occurring with strength & conditioning professionals training tactical athletes?

Trainers spend hours in facilities looking at foot placement, knee tracking and degrees of flexion regarding lifting technique. But, how often do they look at issues such as movement efficiency in running with combat gear, walking while carrying a weapon or disembarking from a vehicle like a tank?

Is there ever any analysis of the techniques tactical athletes must engage in order to get off the floor from a supinated position, post-exercise while in body armor?

The point is that the average trainer does what is easy. And what is easy is to just drop the tactical athlete into the mold of any of the traditional athletic models. In this context, this means models of training based on sports like football, soccer, powerlifting, etc. The tactical athlete is not a collegiate swimmer. The tactical athlete is not a high school soccer star. The tactical athlete is not an Olympic hopeful. Therefore, it is irresponsible for any trainer to use these conventional paradigms to train the tactical athlete.

Let's shift gears.

The stereotype or popular image of the tactical athlete is completely disconnected from the actuality of what this individual has to encompass. Many imagine the tactical athlete has an innate high athletic aptitude. This translates into possessing copious speed, power, endurance, coordination and general fitness.

While it is true most tactical athletes are paid for tasks tied to their level of physical performance — much as professional athletes are -- there is a giant leap being made here. Talent and athletic aptitude are not prerequisites for the tactical athlete in the way they are for the professional athlete.

So what is the real issue here? The real issue is the fact that the majority of trainers approach the tactical athlete assuming a higher-than-average level of coordination, strength, capacity and agility — such as they expect of the collegiate or professional athlete.

This is where the disconnect arises. College and professional athletes have made it to advanced levels of competition, largely based on a culmination of genetic talent and athletic development. This is not the case with the tactical athlete. While many tactical athletes participated in high school athletics (and sometimes even college athletics), it is unreasonable to assume this is representative of the experience of the majority of tactical athletes.

Reflecting back on the physical standards I had to meet to complete basic Army and Special Forces training, I ask myself: "Was it challenging?" And the not very satisfying answer is: "Sometimes."

Another way to ask the question would be: "Was the standard high for the average, American body-type or physical condition?" Again, the answer is not all that appropriate, it is a resounding: "Perhaps."

However, it must also be understood that in the field of physical training, that entrance standards for the military and law enforcement are quite low and unrepresentative of what these jobs typically require of the individual.

Let's play a game. Close your eyes. Wait, don't close your eyes, you won't be able to read.

Rewind your life in your head. Go back to high school or college. Answer the following questions while putting names and faces to each.

1. Which classmates joined the military or law enforcement? Include classmates that simply talked about the prospect in earnest (even if you are not sure they followed through).
2. What kind of people were they?
3. Did they play sports? Did they dominate those sports?
4. Were they athletic in a general sense? Fast? Coordinated? Powerful?
5. Were they social? Confident? Confused? Angry? Scared?
6. Did they seek physical competition because they could easily win? Or, because they enjoyed the challenge?

In answering these questions, I expect you will begin to get a clearer picture of what I hope to focus on in this manual.

In large part, the individuals that come to mind were defined by their mental toughness and motivation to achieve. They were passionate athletes defined by their physical effort and, above all, mental fortitude. And, they were generally people more interested in the challenge than in the ease with which they could surpass the rest of the field.

TIME TO TRAIN

Don't let the final 20% of training ruin 80% of the results.

The above mantra is critical to training the tactical athlete. The meaning is fairly straightforward and is easily applied to strength &

conditioning. However, in my experience, most coaches and trainers are overly concerned with the final 20% of the training and as a result achieve minimal overall improvement.

Most fitness certifications and educational bodies will note that the job of strength & conditioning professionals is to help athletes reach their genetic potential. Through physical training, nutrition and proper recovery, athletes will achieve maximum performance.

This is all fine for the competitive athlete.

For tactical athletes, achieving their genetic potential is NOT the goal. Instead, the need is to focus upon injury prevention, capacity development and functional ranges of movement.

This is an athlete who will compete on

a daily, weekly and annual basis, with rest and de-loading periods occurring irregularly. The level of competition or physical demand is generally not benefited by peaking physical maximums. The key for the TA is typically the ability to sustain the effort over the entire "action" or workday.

If you think this is inaccurate, ask any combat operator or tactical professional: "Do you spend 100% of your physical effort and ability on each movement you perform for the duration of your mission or shift? Or, do you need to reserve 20% in the event the primary plan is unsuccessful?"

Obviously, that is not the mindset a competitive athlete needs to engage. The competitive athlete goes all out for the duration of the competition and then the action is over in a pre-set period of time.

There are no whistles in combat or crisis that signify the end of the mission. The fight continues until the fighting is over. There is no finish line visible from the outset.

Moving on, let's discuss the most critical component of training the tactical athlete: cultural adaptation. Training the TA is more about leadership than fitness knowledge. This is not to suggest that a weak knowledge base is acceptable; rather, the key tenet of success is the ability to demonstrate self-confidence within a leadership role.

This notion may seem elementary and simple commonsense but it is an oft-ignored factor in training. Almost every scenario of physical preparation for the TA is conducted in a group setting or, at minimum, in pairs. The ability of an operator to function as a part of a team is integral to every type of tactical athlete.

Whether the TA is a Marine sniper or an undercover law enforcement officer, missions are rarely, if ever, conducted alone. Therefore, planning and management of the strength & conditioning program must reflect the same operational imperative. Most professionals call this "sport-specific training." I call it "getting it done."

I believe that many who have never served find it difficult to understand military culture. There is a brotherhood that exists that is too difficult to communicate to people without those common experiences.

Note:
Maintaining sets of defined rules that are based upon formal and informal standards help groups achieve goals. These codes of conduct extend throughout professional interactions.

So, how is an individual expected to achieve respect from a military unit (or TA) without possessing the shared experience of suffering through military training and deployment? How do soldiers communicate with civilians who do not even understand military acronyms or contexts?

The answers to these questions are simultaneously very simple and endlessly complex. Coaches and trainers must adopt a durable philosophy: be humble, be confident, and be adaptive. Every environment and scenario is unique. And, having a mindset that makes the process better with each change or stress is essential.

Humility is important to being human. We must be comfortable with small failures and awkward happenings in order to learn and improve. Successful training or teaching is accomplished by connecting mentally and emotionally to the athlete. Therefore, communication becomes the foundation of success.

The science of adaptation to physical stresses creates accomplishment. The cultivation of trust and responsibility to the individual produces success. The balance between the experience of the tactical athlete and the knowledge of the strength & conditioning professional means the creation of an effective program.

Confidence is gained after the correct measure of humility is applied. The strength & conditioning professional needs to command authority and establish leadership through the strength & conditioning process.

Adaptation is difficult. It is tough to build durable systems that get stronger when tested or stressed. The perfect answer does not exist. But I do believe there are some best answers. These are three suggestions for working with and training the tactical athlete:

- Build a strong feedback loop into the team integrations. Whether this occurs through formal weekly reviews or informal daily talks, trainers need to drive an open discussion forum.
- Do not get married to a modality or rigid program. Rigid things break.
- Do not underestimate the power of demonstration. Being able to perform the prescribed movement is important when developing expectations from tactical athletes.

A STRENGTH & CONDITIOING PROGRAM *(with exercise science mixed in)*

Some of the key tenets and ideas to bear in mind during program creation are outlined below. Apply these to your athlete assessment, cycle development and exercise prescription.

Injury prevention through increasing functional range of movement is paramount (remember the 80%/20% mantra). Injury prevention exercise should be engaged in as often as possible -- meaning daily.

Examples of these include:

- Hip bridging and bucking to support ground tactics;
- Wrist flexion and extension;
- Dorsiflexion to support step-down activities:
  - Anaerobic sprints to sustain glycolic work.
  - Chase
- Sprints from a seated position to support vehicle exit.
- Ground-based upper body pushing/ pulling to support suspect detention-related actions.
  - Control and improvement of posture and muscular tone:

- o Most operators suffer from severe hypertonicity and synergistic dominance.
- o Assume all operators are asymmetrically loaded due to the use of tactical equipment for operations (i.e. guns and magazines are asymmetrically loaded on the body).
- Address the forward pelvic tilt that can cause a sway back:
  - o Bring the hips into a neutral position. Pectorals, latissimus dorsi, hip flexors and quadriceps are the big muscles that need to be lengthened, stretched and made healthy.
  - o Strengthening the hamstrings, lower traps and abductors will most effectively increase functional strength.

The TA trainer needs to be able to quickly show the athlete that

quantifiable results are being
achieved. To do this:

- Define your own or unit-specific
  testing with standards at the
  outset.
- Be attentive to formal testing.
  Examine any such required standards
  prior to beginning training. For
  example, the Army PFT is important
  to a given Army commander but may
  not be a good assessment of overall
  physical fitness.
- The ability to identify injury
  prevention in a quantifiable manner
  can be the difference between the
  success and failure of a program.

Rest & Recovery
- Rest is the most critical component
  of the training program.
- Most operators fail to incorporate
  rest and recovery.
- Constant analysis of overtraining is
  necessary.

- Teach recovery techniques: soft
  tissue mobilization and flexibility.

Always remember, the human body is
complex and resilient — it is not
linear and rigid. The greatest impact
a strength & conditioning professional
can make is not science-based — it is
culturally based. Humility, confidence
and adaptability are the cornerstones
that create success.

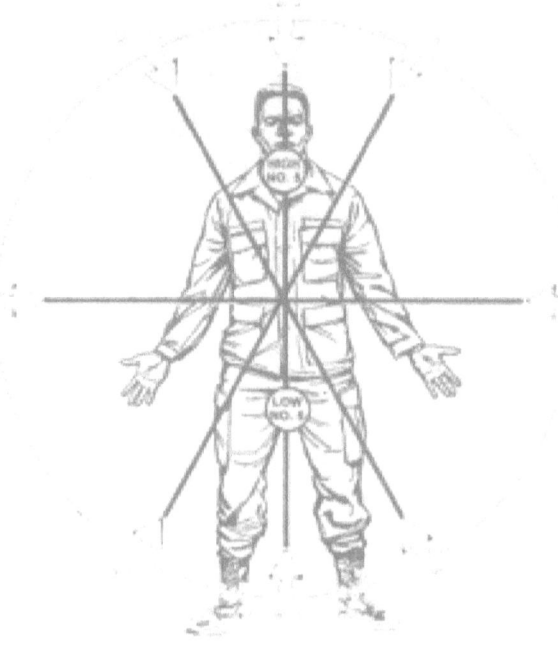

The second step in my tactical fitness methodology is defining a functional movement screen (FMS). There are currently a number of FMS programs out there -- the most popular defined by Gray Cook and Lee Burton. This kind of screening is key to athlete analysis and program construction. The screen helps the trainer better define the athlete, focus the fitness protocol and identify the desired outcome(s).

Create your own FMS!

An FMS should be easily defined, unambiguous and readily duplicated in the training environment. Create a ranking and grading system that documents movement patterns from a logical analysis of normal body function. By screening these patterns, your process should identify those functional limitations and asymmetries that can reduce the effects of physical conditioning and distort body awareness. The process should be a baseline assessment to track the athlete's clinical progress.

The human body includes many joints that generally alternate from mobile to stasis. For example, starting from the ground up, the ankle is highly mobile. The next, proximal joint is the knee, which is considered a stable joint, as flexion and extension are its primary planes of motion. This trend is true throughout almost all of the human body with a few exceptions. It is important to understand this concept when creating an FMS.

While the athlete may be able to complete a given motion, the trainer must consider that it is even more valuable to know whether or not the movement is coming from the right place (i.e. if other muscle groups and joints are being recruited to perform the action).

Note:

The trainer clearly needs to have some basic understanding of anatomy and biomechanics in order to identify dysfunction and proper corrective priority. Any strength & conditioning professional who does not possess this kind of education is not cut out for training and should put down this manual and find a new profession.

Your FMS is an analytical tool. However, the process should not be considered or structured as a predictor of an athlete's ability to excel at any given task. Moreover, the test should not be used as a metric for the comparison of athletes. Athletic or operational success can be developed from the information acquired in the screen, but there has to be a corrective and performance bridge that enables the athlete to get from one to the other. You must be able to take the information collected and transition the athlete appropriately back to full capacity (if injured) or maintain optimal and peak efficiency of movement (if healthy).

The healthy athlete has the greatest likelihood of being able to get through repetitions of training, which in turn enables success.

The ubiquitous adages, "If you're not assessing, you're guessing" and "we don't guess, we gauge" are still important. It is essential to have a qualitative measurement for baseline movement competency that is adaptive and specific to the needs of the tactical athlete. Do not fail to incorporate these into training.

If you take nothing away from my emphasis on the importance of an FMS beyond the understanding that, at minimum, there is an immediate and vital need to transition TAs away from erroneous mindsets such as "no pain, no gain" and "pain is weakness leaving the body."

Pain is a hard-wired, biological mechanism that gives us critical feedback that something needs to change. Pain has the single greatest influence on human movement.

The TA is inherently active and often operates through painful scenarios (mental, emotional and physical). This facet of the job requires mental and emotional toughness to consistently endure the rigors of operation. However, it is the trainer's job to hone the maturity of the tactical athlete.
Athletes must recognize and compartmentalize that strength & conditioning training cannot be executed in the same manner as their professional activities. No matter how tough the soldier, pain will affect physical function and therefore

tactics -- consciously or otherwise. Ignorance is no longer an excuse.

Unfortunately, another common misconception in tactical fitness is the stratification of physical training priority. An industry-wide shift in mindset is in order. Movement quality and proficiency is paramount and should be prioritized.

Second, performance (physical capacity and conditioning) should be emphasized. Lastly, attention to skill acquisition, namely the tactics themselves, and sport-specific training should be considered.

Simply completing the physical task is no longer sufficient. Efficiency and movement mindfulness are more essential. Prioritize the training hierarchy. The screen can be as simple as it needs to be or as complex as the trainer feels necessary. Starting with a simple screen allows for easy implementation in nearly all tactical settings.

Creating an adaptive screen is critical to your success. Embrace the idea that your screen will evolve with your education and experience. So, start with simple assessment tools (i.e. dowels and blocks), but do not be handcuffed to your original concept. Do not be afraid to adapt as you become more skilled.

Your FMS should create a low "barrier to entry" protocol and should possess a complexity that scales as the TA progresses. The screen is meant as a first line of defense to reveal as many potential issues with movement as possible. Let principles of joint-by-joint analysis, regional inter-dependence and nervous system integration, lead to the acquisition of a deeper understanding of the individual.

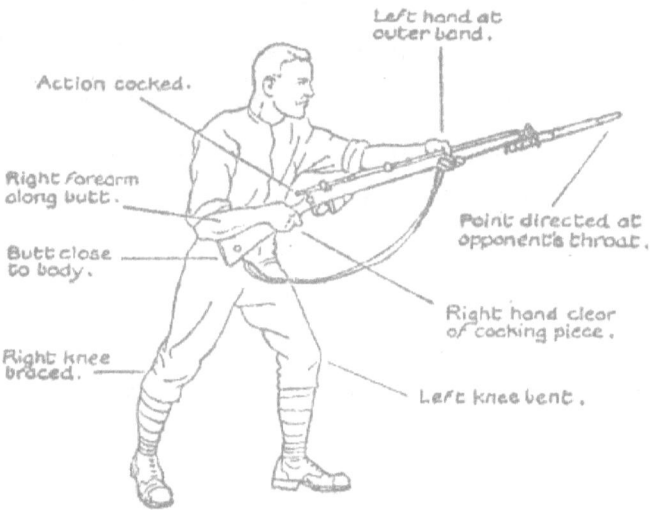

Left hand at outer band.

Action cocked.

Right forearm along butt.

Butt close to body.

Right knee braced.

Point directed at opponent's throat.

Right hand clear of cocking piece.

Left knee bent.

Section 3 - Training Specificity

A friend, co-conspirator and magnificent coach authored this third section. I feel it is best to explain some of the philosophy behind training specificity using his words because, although he is not a tactical athlete, I believe he sincerely understands what is key to achieving real success in this dynamic industry.

I have a good friend who is a former Special Forces operator with combat experience. He once told me that his unit's "mission scope" was that of sub-surface infiltration. He then told me that, as far as he knew, in the history of the U.S. Army, there had not been any assault of this kind, ever. Yet, his team spent countless hours preparing for this "mission"-type when, in reality, what they actually did 95% of the time was drastically different.

I also worked with another group of soldiers who, when asked, reported they spent the majority of their training going on long rucks or runs, only to find that when deployed, they spent the majority of their time in a seated position with an occasional sprint required and almost never went on long marches.

I understand each of these groups needed to be proficient in the skills they were trained in so as to be able to perform their mission scope. But, I believe it would make more sense to allocate training time in accordance with what tactical athletes will most often encounter in the field. At the very least, a more balanced training regimen would be more practical.

Enter the realm of "specificity of training." Specificity of training means the athlete will engage in training stimuli that very closely mimic, if not exactly replicate, the real-time situation for which they are preparing.

The goal is to have the response to the training stimuli meet the physiological requirements of the sport/mission of the athlete with utmost precision. There are many factors to consider, but the following concepts are well supported.
The more similarly training replicates the sport or job duty, the more adequately the participant will be prepared. The greatest improvements in muscle function following training are registered with the modality that most closely matches the actual movement. Training and testing in velocities that are as close to real situations as possible also create opportunities for premium results.

When considering specificity of training for the tactical athlete, one should consider addressing a number of variables before developing a periodized training program. Identifying strength and power needs, energy system requirements, movement types, vulnerabilities to injury, exercise selection, available implements and awareness of the current physical status of the athlete or operator — all these are critical to designing a program that will be effective and safe.

With regard to strength and power production, it is important to first look at how much is needed and in what capacity it will be required. In order to do this, the trainer must investigate the likely loads the particular team may encounter on any mission.

For any given object there is likely a certain weight, distance and method that could potentially be used to move the object. In other words, will the item be pushed, pulled, dragged or carried? In which planes will this occur? Will those methods be employed by one individual or by a team of athletes? What distances are likely to be covered? When dealing with power or force production, will this power be used against another object, person or some other external stimuli?

All these are important considerations that need to be addressed before randomly prescribing exercises to the tactical athlete in training. Exercise selection for strength and power should follow biomechanical specificity to reproduce the same biomechanics and velocities used in combat or in mission-specific tasks.

Programming should also take into account the individual's current status when beginning the training. Knowing the current level of performance, and/or injury status is critical when prescribing specific tasks.

Utilizing the proper energy system for a task at hand is of equal importance. Variables should be manipulated such that the focus is on the primary metabolic pathway and the work-to-rest ratios are as close to those encountered in real life as possible.

In designing a program around energy systems, one must look closely at whether or not the desired training adaptation is being reached. There are many devices that can get the athlete into the desired cardiovascular range for a specified time.

For example, when analyzing a professional hockey player, the trainer would look at which energy systems may be in use and how to modify training to meet those demands. It is common for an NHL forward to skate anywhere between 45 to 75 seconds per shift alternating with 120-165 seconds of rest - as there are typically four offensive lines. This makes the work to rest ratio roughly 1:2.

Of course, this athlete may be closer to 1:1 at certain times in the game; for example, during a power play or toward the conclusion of the game. A player may skate about 7.5 minutes per period; therefore, by the end of the game, the player will have skated roughly 22-23 minutes. Of course, times vary based on position and player, but these are fairly accurate baseline estimates that provide an idea of the specific needs of each. To be as specific as possible, one can break things down further by looking at the type of position. For example, defensemen have a much different role, play longer shifts and have different movement needs.

There are typically three defensive lines in professional hockey, which means there are fewer players at these positions who play longer shifts and have fewer rotations. The ratios may be the same (i.e. 1:1 or 1:2), but the time-on-ice is usually longer for a defenseman, who may average 8.5 minutes per shift and up to 28 minutes per game.

This information can be applied to the players' preseason on ice and dry land training protocol. A typical session on the ice in the preseason may be an hour to an hour and a half with emphasis on breakouts, endurance and over-speed training. And, there may be additional time set aside to address the specific skills of each player.

The team may be on the ice in this capacity for 5-6 days a week. In addition to ice time, the team maintains dry land-based performance training 4-5 days per week to complement efforts on the ice. These sessions tend to run roughly 90 minutes — or the length of a regulation game.

The job of the performance staff serving a hockey team is to examine the minutes played, movements used, work-to-rest ratios, physical limitations and the strength of each player. The expectation is that the coach can create a consistent and effective protocol for each athlete while bearing in mind the team dynamics.

Similarly, this same practice should be employed for the tactical athlete across the spectrum of job specialties. The trainer must look at the unit mission scope, each operator's role within that unit and at each operator's physical capabilities. Further factors to add include execution or duration of deployment, weather, personal equipment load, etc. -- in order to make the training as specific as possible.

Movement is the next variable to be addressed, as noted in the previous section of this handbook. However, the picture is much bigger that purely the concept of movement itself. The coach must consider everything outlined thus far and apply movement-specific exercises based on that information. In other words, it is very important to understand the job and the specific movements necessary to accomplish said job: the velocity, energy systems employed and situations under which the work is performed.

Each tactical group has unique movement needs that must be met. Within the group, each individual has even more specific needs based upon height, weight, injury status and amount of equipment carried. When observing the team during training, the trainer should track and note movement variables.

The activities done daily to complete the tactical job may include movement in multiple planes. This means the task may have a component of movement forward and backward, left and right, and up and down in any combination. Often when this is the case, there is a rotational component to the movement as well.

Try to determine if the TA's movements are compound or single joint. For example, lifting a heavy object from ground to over the head is a good example of a multi-joint movement. A single joint movement may involve performing a repetitive task with a weapons system, machine or other apparatus. Single limb activities present unique strength and core challenges versus double limb ones that are usually easier to integrate.

Note:

Consider that prolonged sitting or standing are also common in tactical positions and require a tremendous amount of postural and posterior chain strength-endurance.

The specific movement can be any combination of the above, but there are necessary factors to be included when developing training regimens including: energy system, velocity, duration and external stimuli.

The trainer should consider if the program addresses all of these variables when looking at movement. Movement in the tactical environment should be addressed much more thoroughly than just confirming that squatting or running is done properly.

Injuries are a common occurrence in athletics as well as in tactical scenarios. For the sake of this discussion, I will address common injuries often sustained during improper training - not injuries that are traumatic in nature.

First, it is necessary to identify injuries that are commonplace within the scope of the protocol in order to be able to program potential fixes for each in a preventative capacity. For example, numerous police departments have reported that vehicle exits in order to engage in pursuit are common scenarios where officers are injured.

In these instances, initially the officers are essentially motionless. They then make an abrupt stop (slam on the brakes), open the door, turn, exit, sprint, pursue and restrain/fight a suspect. Many departments have already begun analyzing the data on this activity and are prescribing exercises to strengthen officer ability to engage in this activity without injury. As a result of this training adjustment, injuries are decreasing.

The point is that the involved departments took data, extracted specific movements related to a common action, defined the conditions under which these movements were executed and developed an appropriate program to reduce these types of injuries. The moral here is: Don't be lazy! It not only leads to inefficient workforce utilization but also increases costs in terms of leave and on-the-job injury expenses.

When observing group training, it is important to know where the areas of vulnerability are and how to correct them. Pre-habilitation specificity can provide a systematic approach to identifying common injuries within a specific sport or tactical profession. In turn, this can then identify appropriate exercises or movement training to minimize their incidence.

Many coaches have already developed a multi-segment method of analyzing this concept for their athletes that has changed the way they construct practice time.

The first step is to manage each athlete's injuries. Next, develop a list of corrective exercises to reduce the likelihood that the given injury will recur. Third, create a program of pre-habilitative exercises to reduce the occurrence of other common training injuries.

It is important to review this with regard to specificity. The coach must take into account the variables of strength and power utilization, energy system development, time, environment, and movement patterns as well as areas of weakness and vulnerability. Then, the coach or trainer must recognize that there are single ideas that overlap in many combinations. The coach must be able to hone in on each of these variables in a focused, progressive and periodized manner.

Integration

Effective training is the key to better performance in any athletic profession. This idea should not be surprising to most coaches. The concept pertains to being fit both physically and mentally. To ensure that an athlete is well prepared before any action, there must be an effective training program in place, one that focuses on the degree of adaptive responses that improve the physical and mental fitness of the athlete.

Of course, programs must focus on volume, intensity and frequency, but they must also maintain a balance through training adaptation that is directly linked to job-specific volume.

Physical development, resilience and

combat readiness are keys to tactical athlete performance in real-time situations. Therefore, the tactical athlete requires training that is more focused on functional job/task specific movements. The program must then promote event readiness while limiting the possibility of injury, and ensuring operators are well prepared both physically and mentally for real-time situations.

Tactical athletes must devote their time and energy to various types of training -- focusing on power, strength, endurance, tactical, speed and agility. Once these types of training have been accomplished and prior to deployment, these athletes also have to engage in the kind of generalized exercise that will support the above, more specific, training.

Keeping the Program Relevant and Adaptive

As noted, there are myriad body types and mission objectives. It is recognized that there is a large scope for training focus. A potential objective of combat training is to build explosive power in order to endure fast-paced, dynamic environments. However, keeping the body and muscles flexible throughout is vital for these types of combat missions. Four phases of development may then be identified, helping keep the programming relevant and adaptive for combat.

The first phase involves foundational training, which aims to make the body more adaptive to strenuous resistance during subsequent training sessions. In this phase, the focus of the training is on the major muscles of the body, ligaments, tendons and various joints, in order to prevent their being injured. Based on the degree of inexperience of a given tactical individual, greater development of foundational strength may be required before moving to the next stage that includes more advanced resistance training such as ballistics, plyometrics, etc.

Even the experienced tactical athlete should spend some time completing the foundational stage of strength training. This is because foundational strength training helps in correcting the muscle imbalance that might occur during deployment.

The second phase is known as the maximum strength phase, where the objective is to make the neuromuscular patterning more adaptive. This phase should always follow the foundational strength-training phase, as it will enable the tactical athlete to gain more strength. Since endurance is also important during combat, maximum strength training helps in building strength for endurance.

The third phase of this type of programming is the explosive, power phase. Combat scenarios tend to move very fast, this calls for more power than just simply lifting loads - as is the case in strength training. If maximum strength is not immediately transformed into special combative power, then the performance of the tactical athlete will not improve to the level it should, as the maximum power output is not converted into combat-specific power. Note that this phase is mainly focused on the overall activities that are always involved in combat-related actions, such as movement and severity.

The last phase involves muscular endurance. Most movements in combat involve the use of a lot of power and explosive action. These movements put a lot of strain on the muscles, calling for muscular endurance training to support the frequency required in combat scenarios. Combat actions need a combination of explosive power and strength to endure — this is a critical balancing act.

Understand that the 4-phase programming referenced here is a general path to explore for a specific subset of tactical athlete. Keep the 80%-20% mantra in mind when defining the maximum strength-to-power phase. Do not become consumed with peaking the tactical athlete's power and forget that success is measured by injury prevention and the achievement of functional movement.

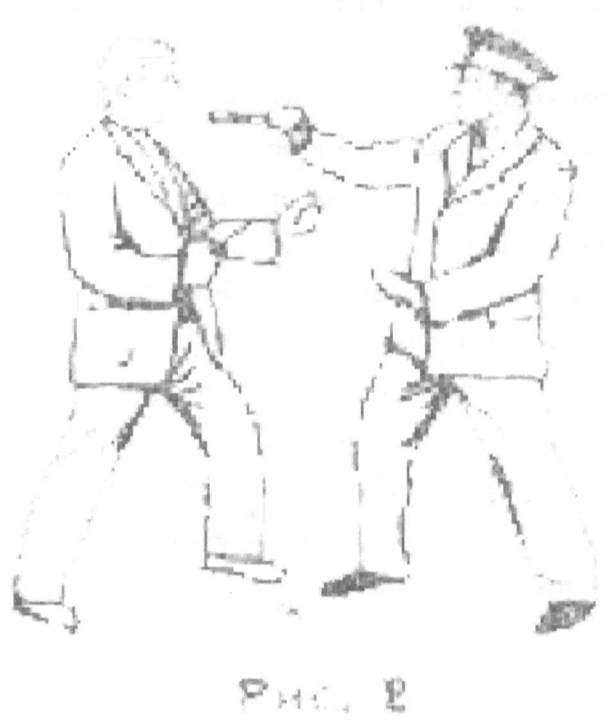

Рис. 2

Performance parameters are based on balancing out the emotional, mental and physical aspects of the tactical athlete. All three of these components depend upon a regular intake of nutrients in order to function at an optimal level. The body and mind become healthy, physically and emotionally, when regular exercise, balanced nutrition and the proper intake of supplements are all components of the daily practice of the athlete.

Anyone in the strength & conditioning industry will agree that nutrition is the most critical and complex component driving performance. The TA must fuel the mind and body. Necessary adaptations to environmental changes require complete attention to mental, physical and emotional states.

While this manual does not examine the

science behind performance nutrition -
- the fitness industry is saturated
with programs that cover this -- it
<u>will</u> assert a philosophy that is
focused on identifying and correcting
the general malaise regarding the
nutrition-coaching relationship.

I am not a nutritionist or dietician.
Therefore, I will make this section
relatively short, looking only briefly
into the science of the industry.
Remember, this document is a
manifesto, not a medical journal -- or
even a technical commentary!

First, a call to action. Do not be
lazy in your education, philosophy or
application of programming. Trainers
are immersed in a sea of propaganda
and distortion that provide easy ways
to ignore our knowledge deficiencies
and simply credit a variety of
unsubstantiated sources.

There is good information out there;

however, many times that good information is buried by the overwhelming powers of marketing and brand appeal. Recycling old material, over-simplifying biology and re-heating old ideas, all these stale concepts keep the multi-billion dollar diet and nutrition industry alive. Fitness retailers and lazy professionals count upon the ignorance and laziness of consumers to sell the "next great product." Get over your own ego, get educated and do right by your customer/client.

It is necessary to adopt a sturdier philosophy to move forward. The tactical fitness industry needs to embrace the idea that every athlete is unique and requires attention to detail when prescribing nutrition and strength protocols. Do not get caught in rigid plans. The human body is an amazing and complex organism — treat it accordingly. Do not simply defer to simplistic programming. Strive to be better than that.

Many in the field are diligently working to improve the understanding of the human body and the optimal/necessary adaptations it must engage in to best deal with its environment. We should be humbled by our ignorance, not threatened by it. We should be inspired by the potential that exists, not afraid of the battles we must fight.

True, we have become a culture driven by studies and acute statistical analysis. We get so focused upon the principal of 10,000 hours of practice and making the athlete an expert that we forget that each body is different. We must underscore the principle that practice doesn't make perfect; perfect practice … makes perfect. And, perfection includes thoroughly analyzing the athlete's unique metabolic and nutritional needs. Both athletes and tactical fitness professionals must adopt a philosophy that demands constant evaluation and open-mindedness toward new ideas that potentially upset popular culture. This idea is extraordinarily demanding, but it is the best path forward. Everyone falters and occasionally fails — be strong enough to keep moving forward.

To return to the beginning: Every day, tactical athletes face physical, mental and emotional stresses that can catch them by surprise. The question is: "Can they utilize the resources their training provides them to adapt, perform and thrive?"

The human digestive system has not had any major changes in a very long time. However, the volume and variety of diets and nutritional programs suggest this system is in a constant state of evolution — an idea that is patently false. The body has always been able to use the nutrition found in regularly available, "normal" food, to fuel the maximal physical, mental and emotional energy levels needed for peak performance and everyday living.

There is no magic nutritional bullet that will catapult athletes to optimal strength and performance.

It makes sense to avoid foods with additives and chemicals — these are clearly not natural. Defining what is unhelpful or not necessary is a great place to begin.

One must acknowledge that performance-enhancing drugs (PEDs) will impact performance. However, the potential, long-term damage these do is almost impossible to calculate or measure. Enough said.

My experience as an athlete and coach has led me to accept a fairly simple idea. The human body needs essential proteins, essential fats and essential amino acids. There is a reason these all include the word "essential." I have never heard of an "essential carbohydrate." So, while I am not suggesting that carbohydrates do not have a place in the athlete's diet — I personally think they are delicious — I just do not understand the thinking of some coaches that it makes sense to load up endurance athletes with high levels of carbs.

Stop it!

Instead of launching more attacks on foods or supplements, let me just list the key takeaways that guide my philosophy.

1. When it comes to proper nutrition, there is no one-size-fits-all approach.
2. Nutrition is difficult; it takes discipline. Work hard at it.

3. To gain strength and muscle, approach meals and nutrition with the same intensity you approach physical training.

4. Be humble - continue to learn.

5. Think, adapt and overcome.

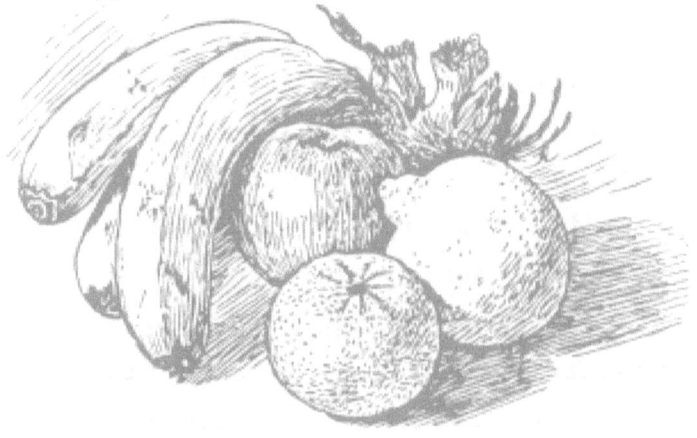

Section 5 - Assessment & Selection

The assessment and selection of strength & conditioning coaches is an issue that profoundly impacts the entire industry. The major impact it has is not universally recognized; however, it is in fact steering the direction of the whole industry.

Since the tactical athlete requires special programming attention, for all of the reasons outlined previously, it is critical to hold to a higher standard those chosen to guide TA physical conditioning programs. Many strength & conditioning professionals are frustrated by TA-specific factors such as deployments and irregular schedules. This frustration is compounded by all the other difficult training variables: athletic aptitude, injuries, education, motivation and available equipment.

Unqualified and poorly evaluated

coaches are filling many strength & conditioning positions within the tactical fitness industry. The blame for this is shared. Hiring managers, recruiters, coaches, retailers and, of course, tactical athletes themselves must take responsibility for this failure. If such training were a new or evolving field, ignorance would be a valid excuse. However, the tactical fitness industry is not new, novel or even underrepresented.

I hope I haven't lost anyone because now I'm going to turn up the heat. This one aspect of tactical fitness fuels most of my dissatisfaction with the industry. While the strength & conditioning coach is the user interface, administrators and recruiters are the engine of laziness and misinformation. Therefore, I hope to motivate a "from the ground up" movement to reorganize and reshape those that are corrupting the field.

Generally, when I am making a point, I will use the Special Forces soldier as the manifestation of the standard tactical athlete. I do not know everything about Special Forces. As a matter of fact, I know very little; I only served for 8 years.

I am writing this handbook from a place of empathy and anger. Unless you have lived the life, it is difficult to comment on it. You can watch all the Rambo movies, Discovery Channel and Nat. Geo. Special Forces documentaries but without direct experience, it is hard to really grasp the experience in depth. (But if you have a few hours to spend, "Two Weeks in Hell" on Discovery is the one I think does the best job.)

People have to be out of their minds to believe a college degree in Exercise Science, a Certified Strength & Conditioning Specialist credential, and experience limited to working with professional or college athletes, qualifies them to train tactical athletes.

Even working with Olympic-level athletes does not mean a trainer can comprehend the unique training requirements of the tactical athlete. The reason for this is that each of these athlete types is already possessed of a degree of athletic ability — or the individual would not be competing at the high school, college or Olympic level.

The skill set required to train the tactical athlete is unique and complicated. The tactical athlete is an individual who is not an athlete first but rather, an individual choosing to pursue a complex career path that, in addition to the rigors of the job, requires the acquisition of a degree of athletic ability, usually very specific in nature.

It is ridiculous, and frankly, offensive to a certain degree, to insinuate that someone can easily make the jump from competitive athlete training to that for tactical athletes without obtaining additional education or experience.

In addition, there is the matter of pay. The financial compensation offered for tactical training positions is substantially lower than that paid in the training industry as a whole. By failing to offer competitive salaries, the tactical training industry also sells its athletes short as it is attracting a less experienced, less motivated applicant.

The question is then obvious. Who is the best fit for tactical fitness and how do we attract that "type" to the field? Let's begin with a clean slate. Which characteristics are we seeking? We need to examine the job description and redefine the selection process.

While I feel the scope of positions and required characteristics is too large to address in this handbook, I will list a few ideas to consider.

- The expectations a given tactical unit will have for a strength & conditioning coach will vary based on the activities of the unit. Defining these expectations should include an open discussion among both administrators and recruits/personnel.
- Are there specific personality types that will be better fits for a particular unit? Is strong leadership a requirement of all such units?
- Should the coach have to meet certain physical requirements? Tactical athletes may have more difficulty — than, for example, competitive athletes in high school

or college settings -- in absorbing advice and instruction from a coach they perceive as unable to engage in the prescribed activities.

- Should a coach be expected to exhibit a high level of interest and appreciation for the tactical fitness field? Again, tactical athletes — people consistently facing the possibility that they will have to put their lives on the line — should not have to be coached by an individual who feels the job is unfulfilling, a "lesser" career or not requiring of the full range of trainer ability.
- Is the experience presented by a given applicant truly applicable to the intricacies of the tactical training field?

Here are a few questions, categories and ideas that may help guide a new, integrated process for hiring tactical fitness professionals:

1. Program Implementation Strategy
   a. How will you, as the trainer, convince tactical athletes you possess the skills to help them improve in their chosen field?
   b. To whom, in the program, will you speak first? (This allows you, the interviewer, to understand the applicant's thought process regarding how to integrate into an existing program.)
   c. Do you have a tailored plan that specifically addresses training the tactical athlete?
2. Program Philosophy
   a. What are the program's core concepts, tactical analytics and deliverable outcomes measures?
   b. Are you applying football athlete training practices to the training of Mission Specific tactical athletes? What is the specific purpose of the program structure you propose? Prove the value of your program to the standard tactical athlete.

      c. Which tools will you incorporate to increase the avoidance of injury and -- in all seriousness -- the survival chances of these athletes?

3. Scientific Design
      a. Explain your training process for: energy systems, motor development, biomechanical design and Mission Specific conditioning.
      b. Is your science correct?

4. Performance-Based Interview Questions
      a. What is your situational experience?
      b. Define your:
          i. Problem-solving approach
         ii. Group interaction methods
       iii. Communication skills
        iv. Leadership ability

5. Physical Fitness Proficiency
      a. Tactical athletes require coaches/trainers who can engage in the prescribed activities

themselves. Please demonstrate a prescribed technique.

b. Have you taken the physical fitness test for this tactical unit? What was your score?

c. How is your presentation? Are you believable in the role of tactical athlete trainer? Very subjective but definitely a question the right candidate can easily answer.

6. Require Face-to-Face Interviews

Regarding #6, the difference between a candidate on paper and a candidate in front of you is remarkable. The side note to this is: People are not always "straightforward" on résumés.

In 2011, we first started seeing job postings seeking strength & conditioning professionals to work with Special Operations soldiers. These posting were vague, confusing and required very little education and/or experience.

Special Forces soldiers are held to the highest standards. Why should civilian contractors get a free pass? There is no real selection process, just a list of accepted credentials. What kinds of committee are setting up these standards?

By the end of 2012, nearly a dozen staffing companies were sourcing personnel for such government positions. The general field was not a new business but the staffing companies had no idea what was required of the tactical athlete trainer.

Consequently, the system saw huge turnover with coaches and little efficacy in programs. Not surprising, if you don't have a rigorous screening system, you can't be expected to achieve any level of success.

Which brings us to my last point of contention — success metrics. What constitutes a successful strength & conditioning program? That's a good question. Recall the 80%-20% mantra. This field is not focused on maximizing the genetic potential of the athlete. It is focused on keeping the soldier injury free and physically capable of using the prescribed mission equipment successfully.

More specifically, creating metrics that measure for maximal, physical effort makes no sense in the tactical athlete-training arena. Max push-up, max squat and max sprint efforts are an ineffective gauge of efficacy here. It may look good on a report and garner a manager a promotion but it in no way measures the potential for success of the soldier in the field.

I propose introducing the concept of patience into the defining of metrics. Carefully consider injury rates in respect to training and operational deployments and overlay that data on training protocols. That kind of examination takes time. Most people know the signs and symptoms of overtraining and lack of rest — they manifest in a variety of ways and over the long term. It is unacceptable to tolerate a high level of adrenal fatigue and overuse injuries as just the expected consequence of being a tactical operator.

Flat standards for movement are key and cannot be ignored. For example, all combat soldiers should be able to drag a 150 lb. weight for 50 ft. in order to prove combat worthiness. This is not a standard to be scaled for gender, weight, age or athletic aptitude. The athlete must pass or fail — there is no score, just pass or fail. This is because a soldier must be able to drag another soldier out of harm's way. That is a simple fact of combat and a simple requirement of the

combat tactical athlete. You can't
say in the field: "I get a special
accommodation for that."

To the administrator and hiring
mangers:

Have a process that integrates a quick
feedback loop with units, coaches and
educators. Be flexible. Be humble.

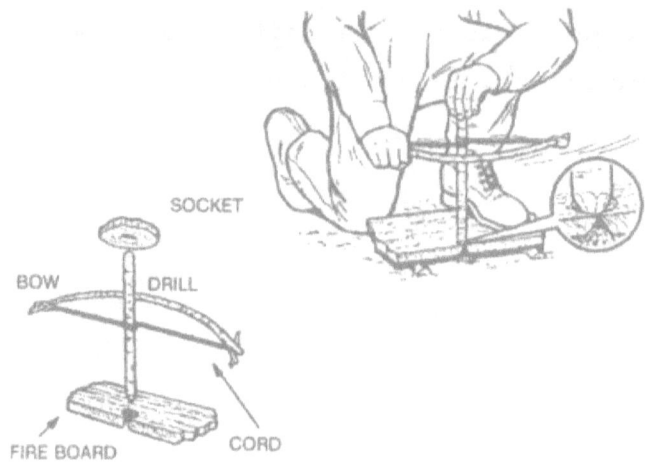

SOCKET

BOW   DRILL

FIRE BOARD   CORD

Section 6 - Closing Thoughts

Dear Thoughtful Athletes and Conditioning Aficionados,

This document is the beginning, the beginning of a discussion that should sharpen our perspective and strategy on training the tactical athlete and shaping the industry as a whole.

First, I want to restate the key tenets of my paradigm.

Humility is obviously important to most things relating to interactions between humans. However, many strength & conditioning professionals forget that the key to successful training is connecting sincerely to their athletes. It is not the science of adaptation to physical stresses that creates champions; it is the cultivation of trust and responsibility to the team, individual or goal that makes the difference.

Therefore, it is the responsibility of the strength & conditioning professional to understand that there is always a *quid pro quo* that correctly balances the experience of the tactical athlete and that of the strength & conditioning professional to create an effective program.

Confidence is projected after the correct measure of humility is applied. Commanding authority and establishing one's leadership under the banner of "subject matter expert" is a delicate balance. Do not be arrogant and do not be submissive. There is no formula to achieving this balance. You just know when you have done it.

Remember a few key things about the tactical athlete. First, most possess a "Type A" personality and are generally used to functioning with high levels of autonomy in high-stress situations. These athletes are physically and mentally tough individuals that have made a living being tougher that the competition. Their mental and emotional fortitude is compounded with generally high physical pain thresholds -- which can often be their greatest asset.

Adaptability is the cornerstone for any worthwhile strength & conditioning program. Out of necessity, tactical athletes are a very cohesive group. We never want to isolate or remove an athlete from the group, if it's possible to avoid. Altering the group dynamic may give rise to dissatisfaction or resentment in the marginalized individual.

Though there are formal rank structures within a tactical unit, the strength & conditioning professional should also identify informal leaders within the group in order to better manage and execute the programming.

Lastly, **communication** is paramount to success. The talent and success of a coach and athlete will never be realized without a foundation of effective communication. Do not be rigid in how you communicate. Some individuals learn well with verbal input, others do better with written instruction, and many achieve greater success through viewing demonstrations. Discover that coach-to-athlete connection. Understand it is a process and hone that connection at every opportunity.

This paradigm shift requires an honesty and sincerity that may make a lot of people uncomfortable. Guess what? Life is often uncomfortable. We need to better understand our strengths and weaknesses both as coaches and as athletes.

This deep honesty is the foundation of specificity as we train the mind and body of the tactical athlete. This perspective is a living idea; therefore, we must constantly evaluate, analyze and adapt our programming so it can remain vital, challenging and productive.

This document is not the ultimate answer — it is a system. We get closer to answers by identifying what does not work and offering new ideas to address those failures. Once we commit to a rigid, black and white policy, we are doomed. Defining training processes through superlatives or finite statements is irresponsible.

Our solution is *via negativia*: a philosophy that embraces the idea that stripping away that which we understand to be bad helps us get closer to that which is good. No perfect solution exists to training the tactical athlete. However, robust systems that gain strength from

mistakes afford us better
opportunities for progress and
success.

Life is a war of attrition. We fight
and fight until the body fails — then
we somehow find the courage and
strength to stand up and fight some
more. In the end, we can only hope
that we made each effort count.

Thank you for reading.

Sincerely,
Derek Zahler

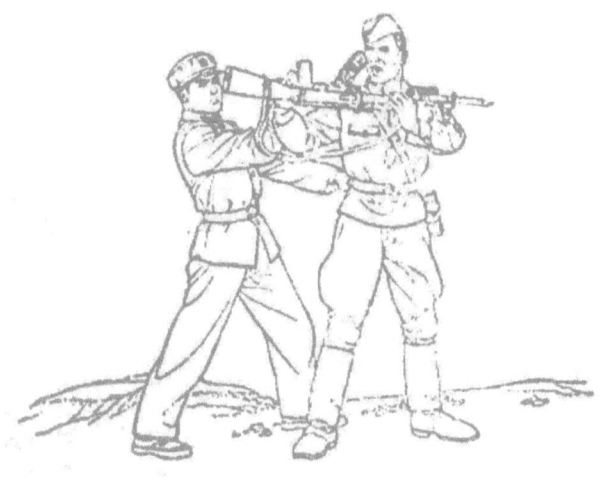